A Healthy view towards Sanitation in our daily life

Thesis on Hygiene and Salubrity June 2014

The Course is indeed very informative and helpful lectured at Access Vocational Education School of Riverside School Board, St Lambert Quebec. It is best for the student who decides to further their career in housekeeping with a touch of deep hygienical procedures and safety. Very descriptive information are being provided about the division of the work.

The expectations after completing this course has changed due to the growing population in size and ethinicity.

To feel at ease in the field of work and understand the core subject of the course so that it is done effectively and efficiently with good understanding of peers.

As I was already dealing with hygiene at my own home and my surrounding area, it was not too difficult to understand the concept of the subject, but I just needed a deeper knowledge for the understanding of how to deal with germs and prevention of infections in a health care environement.

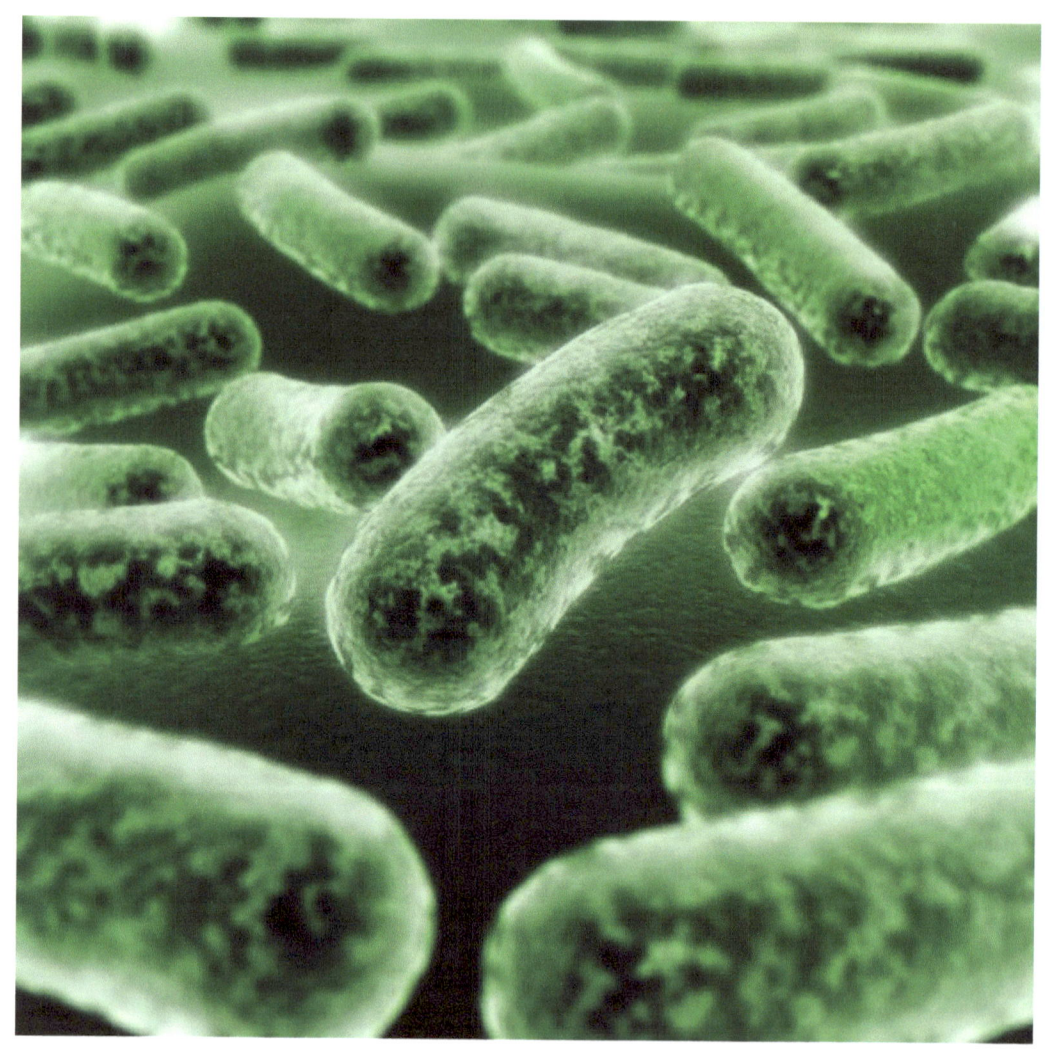

Ranking list of Best Health Care

Canada 30

Mauritius 84

USA 37

Hospital infections are very high!!!

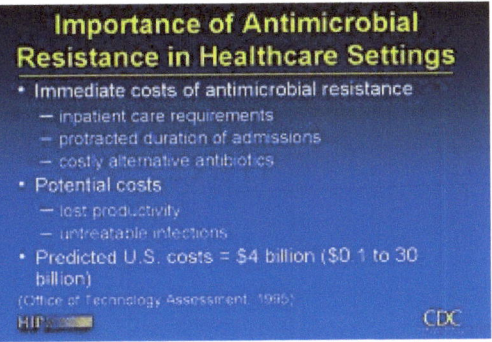

Money Handling can be very infectious full of bacteria and dirty job it can do, corruption.

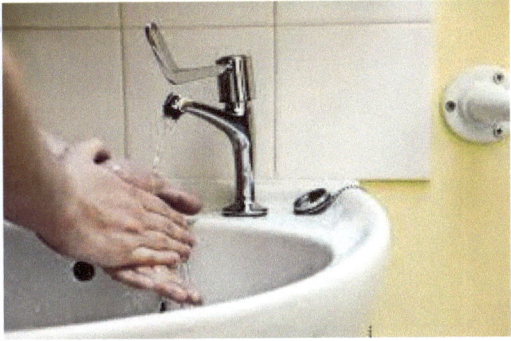

Learn to better cure

Study to better cure

Research to better cure

Means of transmissions

Droplets: Mucous

Airborne: Germs in the air

Secretions: perspirations

Excretions: fecal, urine, vomit

Vehicle: furniture, surfaces

Contact: physical

Ports of Entry are: Nose, Eyes, Nails, Skin and Mouth

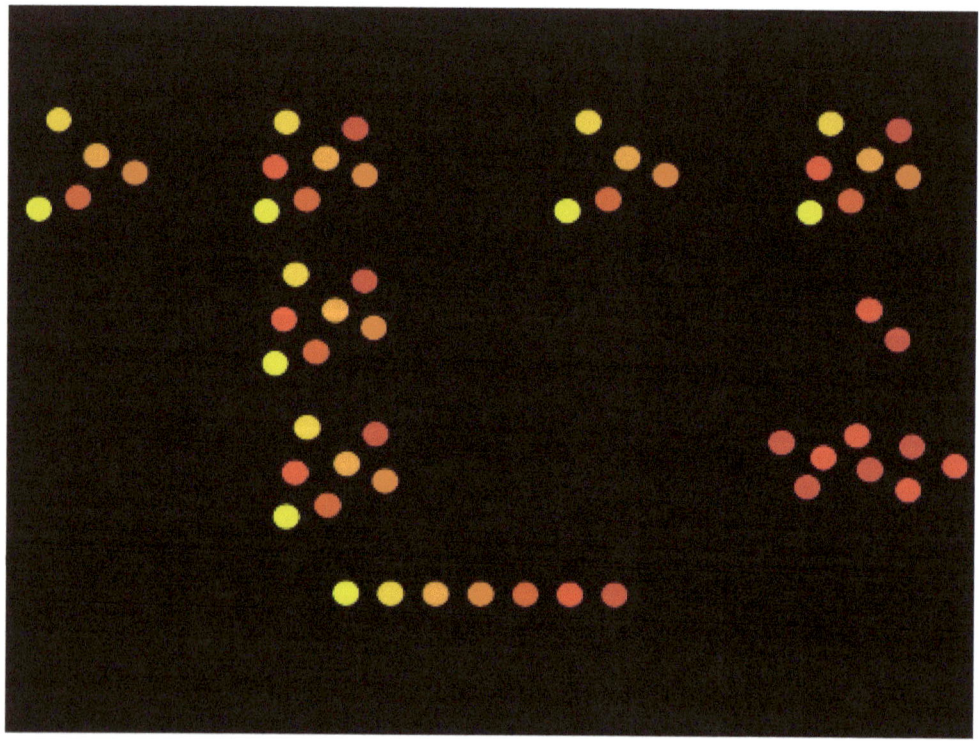

Always wash hands as soon as you feel they are dirty.

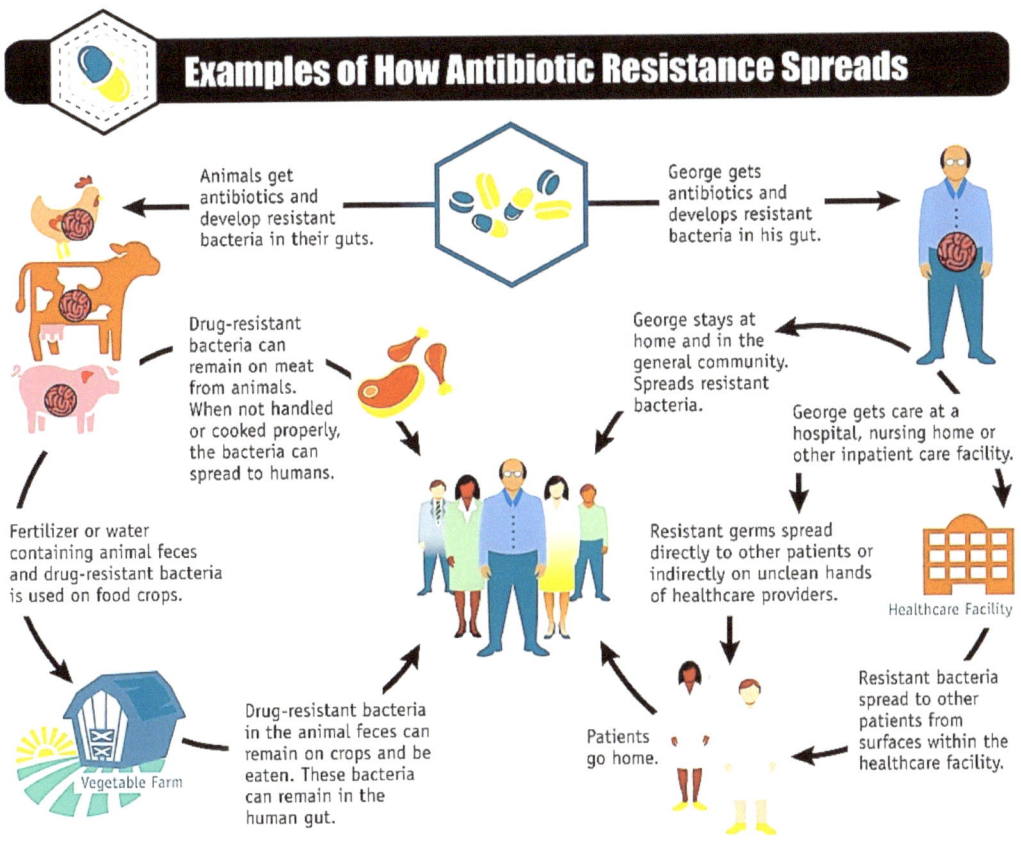

Examples of How Antibiotic Resistance Spreads

Animals get antibiotics and develop resistant bacteria in their guts.

George gets antibiotics and develops resistant bacteria in his gut.

Drug-resistant bacteria can remain on meat from animals. When not handled or cooked properly, the bacteria can spread to humans.

George stays at home and in the general community. Spreads resistant bacteria.

George gets care at a hospital, nursing home or other inpatient care facility.

Fertilizer or water containing animal feces and drug-resistant bacteria is used on food crops.

Resistant germs spread directly to other patients or indirectly on unclean hands of healthcare providers.

Healthcare Facility

Vegetable Farm

Drug-resistant bacteria in the animal feces can remain on crops and be eaten. These bacteria can remain in the human gut.

Patients go home.

Resistant bacteria spread to other patients from surfaces within the healthcare facility.

Simply using antibiotics creates resistance. These drugs should only be used to treat infections.

Colonized

Carrier of infectious agent without presenting any symptoms

Infected

Person subjected to an attack with clinical manifestations

Antibiotic Resistance Keeps Increasing

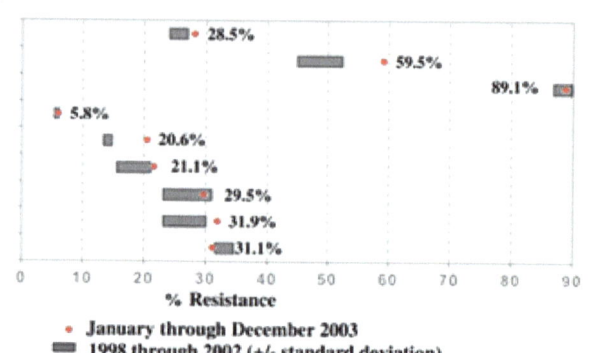

Selected antimicrobial-resistant pathogens associated with nosocomial infections in intensive care unit (ICU) patients, comparison of resistance rates from 2003 with 1998–2002, NNIS System

	% increase in resistance (2003 vs 98-02)
Vancomycin/enterococci 28.5%	12%
Methicillin/*S. aureus* 59.5%	11%
Methicillin/CNS 89.1%	1%
3rd Ceph/*E. coli* 5.8%	0%
3rd Ceph/*K. pneumoniae* 20.6%	47%
Imipenem/*P. aeruginosa* 21.1%	15%
Quinolone/*P. aeruginosa* 29.5%	9%
3rd Ceph/*P. aeruginosa* 31.9%	20%
3rd Ceph/*Enterobacter* spp. 31.1%	−6%

% Resistance

- January through December 2003
- 1998 through 2002 (+/- standard deviation)

Am J Infect Control. 2004;32:470-485.

Adaptation is likely to be an important determinant of the success of many pathogens, for example when colonizing a new host species, when challenged by antibiotic treatment, or in governing the establishment and progress of long-term chronic infection.

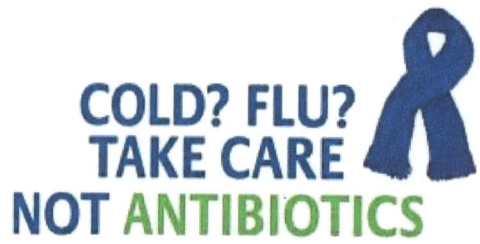

COLD? FLU? TAKE CARE NOT ANTIBIOTICS

A European Health Initiative

Pathogens face a hostile and often novel environment when infecting a new host, and adaptation to this environment can be critical to a pathogen's survival. The genetic basis of pathogen adaptation is in turn important for treatment, since the consistency with which therapies succeed may depend on the extent to which a pathogen adapts via the same routes in different patients.

Difference between a dream which is the result of unconscious rooted feelings which acts as support to the human beliefs and the dormant bacteria which requires a potential host to become a harmful pathogen. They are both actions of the mind and body resulting which are of potential threat to Health.

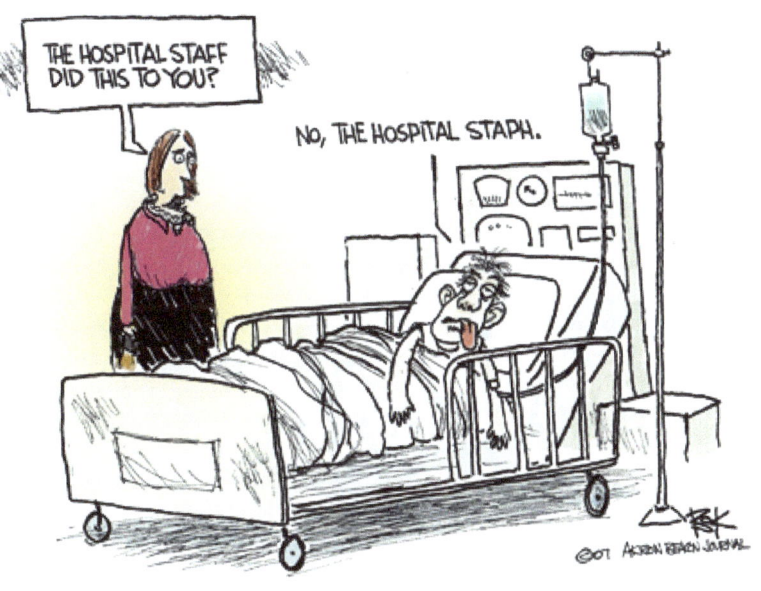

Micro-organisms are organic livings things which becomes pathogens when they are harmful and infectious.

Bacteria is one of the sequence through which germs develop. Some are mutant so they either decrease or increase in their spreading intensity of diseases into epidemic and pandemics.

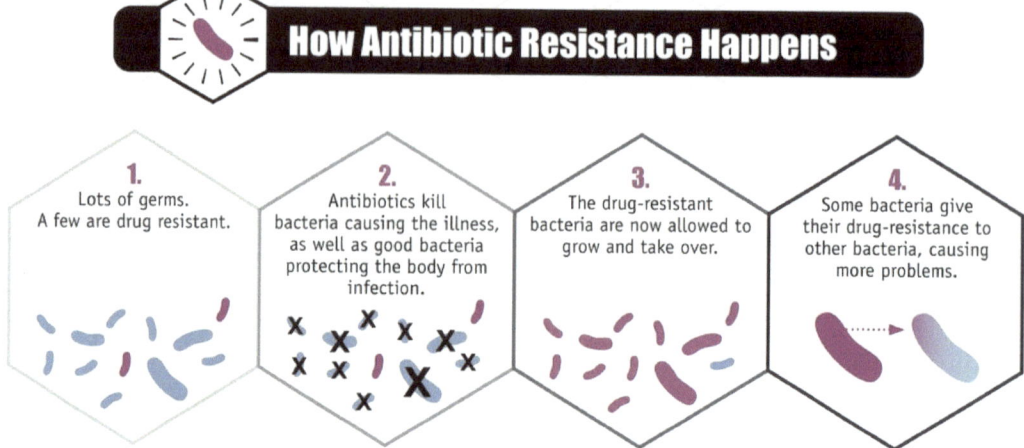

How Antibiotic Resistance Happens

1.
Lots of germs.
A few are drug resistant.

2.
Antibiotics kill bacteria causing the illness, as well as good bacteria protecting the body from infection.

3.
The drug-resistant bacteria are now allowed to grow and take over.

4.
Some bacteria give their drug-resistance to other bacteria, causing more problems.

Survival conditions for bacteria

Oxygen, darkness and humidity

Anti-biotics can lead to Cell Deaths

List of pollutions
Soil, airborne,noise, smell, light and radioactivity.

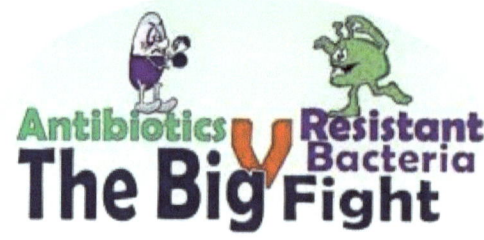

Programmed cell death

Programmed cell death (PCD) is the deliberate suicide of an unwanted cell in a multicellular organism.

In contrast to necrosis, which is a form of cell death that results from acute tissue injury and provokes an inflammatory response, PCD is carried out in a regulated process that generally confers advantages during an organism's life cycle.

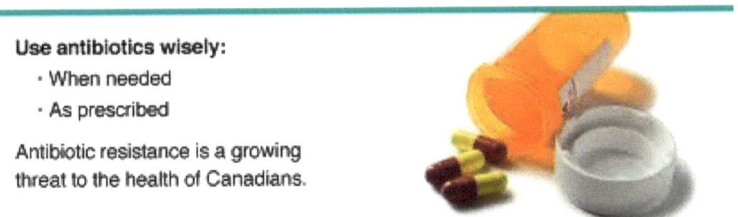

Use antibiotics wisely:
- When needed
- As prescribed

Antibiotic resistance is a growing threat to the health of Canadians.

Traditionally, programmed cell death (PCD) is associated with eukaryotic multicellular organisms. However, recently, PCD systems have also been observed in bacteria. Here we review recent research on two kinds of genetic programs that promote bacterial cell death. The first is mediated by *mazEF,* a toxin–antitoxin module found in the chromosomes of many kinds of bacteria, and mainly studied in Escherichia coli. The second program is found in *Bacillus subtilis,* in which the *skf* and *sdp* operons mediate the death of a subpopulation of sporulating bacterial cells. We relate these two bacterial PCD systems to the ways in which bacterial populations resemble multicellular organisms.

Figures

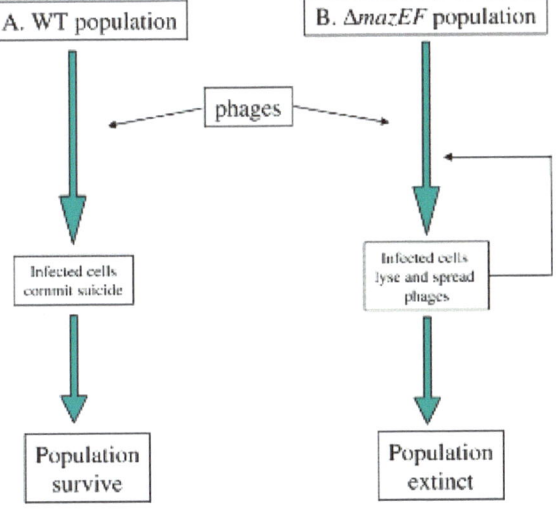

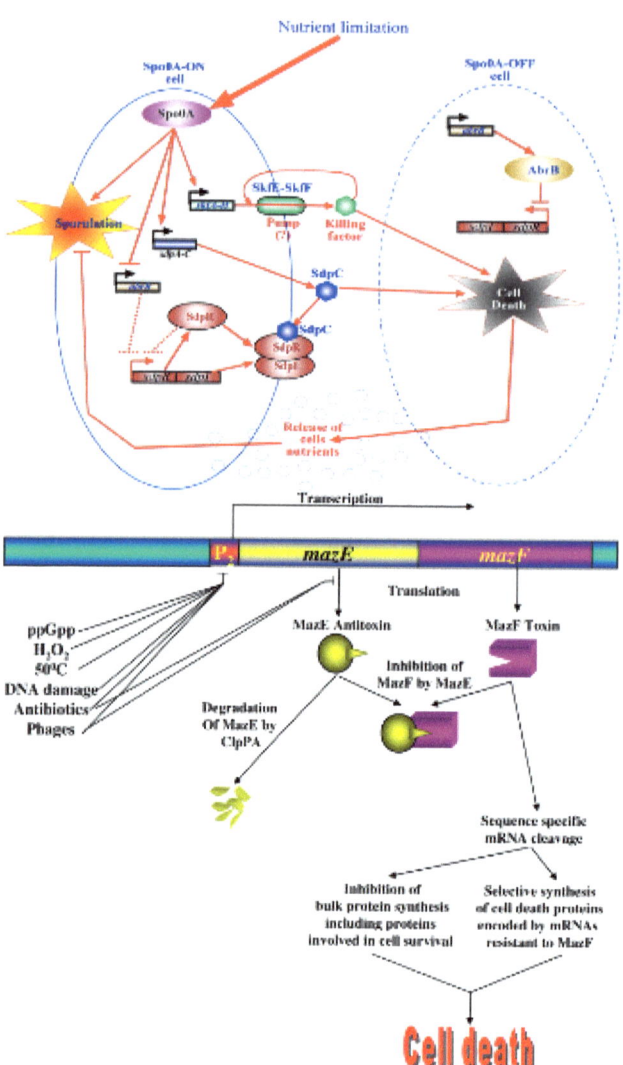

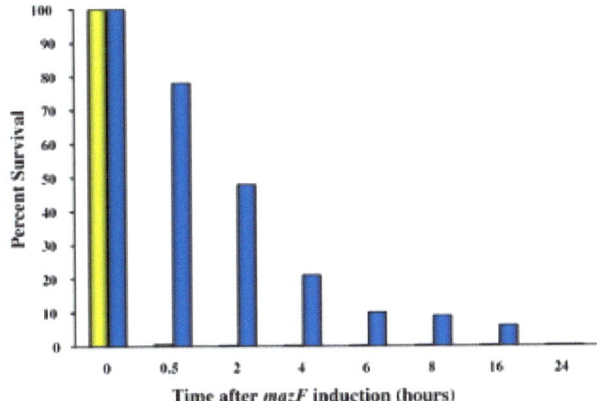

A.

Percent Survival vs. Time after *mazF* induction (hours)

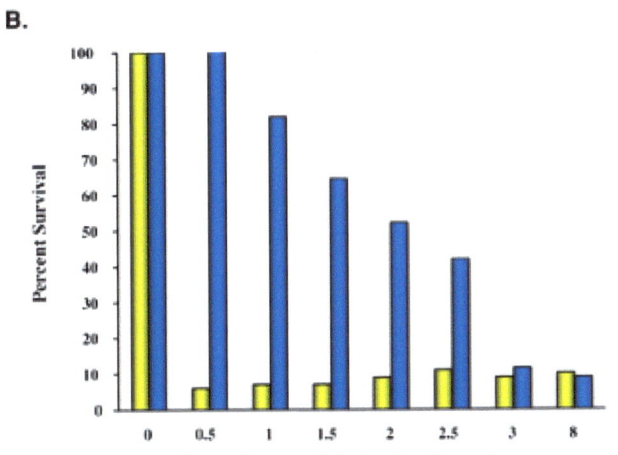

B.

Percent Survival vs. Time after *mazF* induction (hours)

Organism Strain	Protein Hits to E. coli K 12 (Sequenced Wild-Type MG1655)	MazE			MazF		
		Accession Number	Percent Identity	Percent Similarity	Accession Number	Percent Identity	Percent Similarity
Escherichia coli strain K12-MG1655	–	b2781	100	100	b2782	100	100
		b4224	12	34	b4225	31	51
Escherichia coli strain O157:H7 EDL933	10,298	Z4088	100	100	Z4089	100	100
		Z5406	12	56	Z5406	36	52
Salmonella typhimurium LT2 strain SGSC1412	8,648	–	ND	ND	–	ND	ND
Pseudomonas aeruginosa strain PAO1	7,601	–	ND	ND	–	ND	ND
Agrobacterium tumefaciens strain C58 UWash	6,626	Atu0839	10	54	Atu0940	39	53
Bacillus anthracis strain Sterne	5,404	–	ND	ND	BA5040	31	48
Bacillus subtilis strain 168	4,735	–	ND	ND	Bs4b466	33	48
Bacillus halodurans strain C-125	4,499	BH1178	41	64	BH1711	54	48
Listeria monocytogenes strain 4b F2365	3,395	LMOF2318_p1M02_0030	27	49	LMOF2365_0948	33	48
Enterococcus faecalis strain V583	3,121	EFA0072	15	51	EFA0071	31	54
		–	ND	ND	EF3262	36	55
		–	ND	ND	EF3853	30	52
		–	ND	ND	EF3835	31	67
Clostridium perfringens strain 13	2,957	–	ND	ND	CPE0290	26	58
		–	ND	ND	POP58	20	47
Staphylococcus aureus strain Mu50	1,657	–	ND	ND	SA1673	36	48
Deinococcus radiodurans strain R1	3,368	DR0416	45	63	DR0417	44	51
		–	ND	ND	DR0662	29	58
Mycobacterium tuberculosis strain CDC1551	3,461	–	ND	ND	MT2868	41	54
		–	ND	ND	MT1992	20	43
		–	ND	ND	MT2048	36	53
Neisseria meningitidis strain serogroup A Z2491	2,191	–	ND	ND	NMA0400	39	58
Leptospira interrogans strain serovar lai 56601	2,342	LA1780	32	51	LA1781	44	56
Neisseria meningitidis strain MC58	2,119	NMG0914	25	51	NMBV2	31	52
		–	ND	ND	NMB2008	34	58
Neisseria gonorrhoeae FA1090 (Oklahoma)	1,897	NG00317	45	74	NG00316	38	69
Streptococcus mutans strain UA159	1,333	SMU.173	33	49	SMU.173	30	51
		SMU.1786c	17	50	–	ND	ND
Bartonella henselae strain Houston-1	1,425	BH09350	26	63	BH07050	33	51
Rickettsia felis strain URRWXCal2	1,058	–	ND	ND	RF_1543	34	48

The presence of E. coli K12 MazE and mazF homologs in various bacteria was determined by Blast search (threshold of p-value = 1) using the genomic databases of TIGR Comprehensive Microbial Resource Web site (http://cmr.tigr.org/tigr-scripts/CMR/CmrHomePage.cgi). The bacteria are arranged by the number of protein hits between them and E. coli strain K12 MG1655, signifying the homology of the bacteria.

ND, not detected.

DOI: 10.1371/journal.pgen.0030002.t001

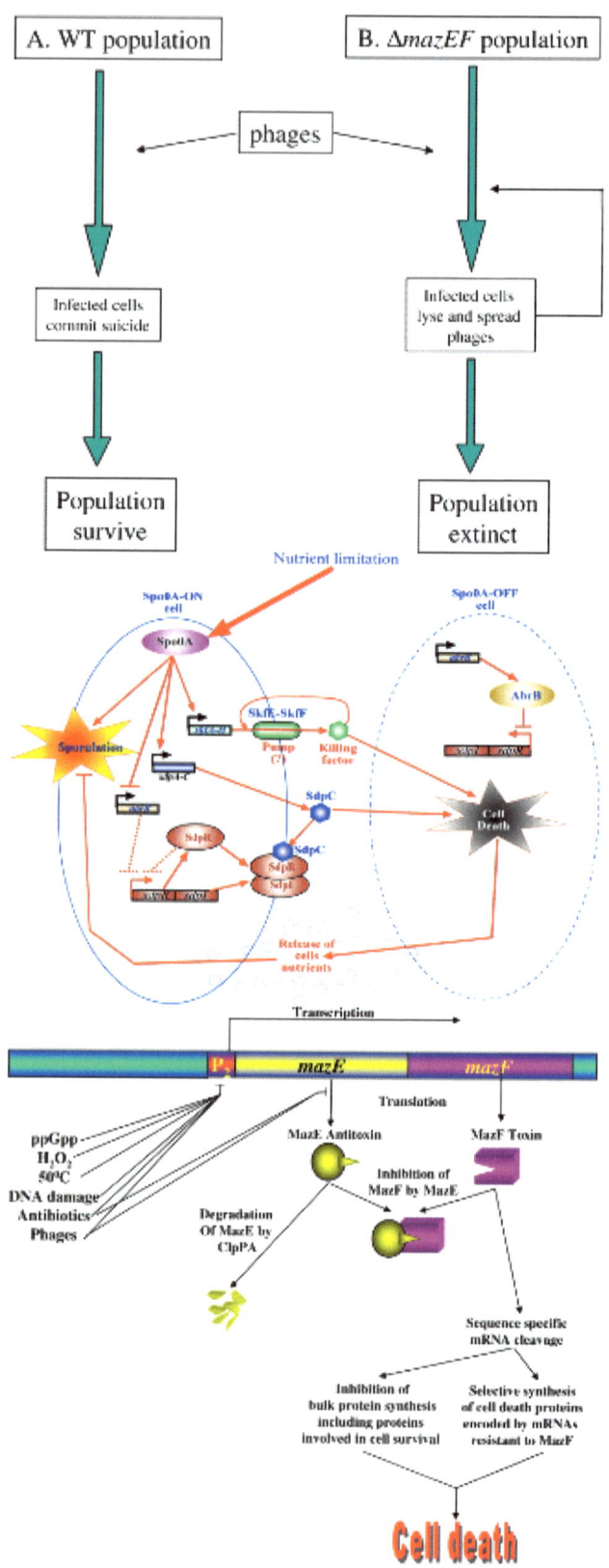

A.

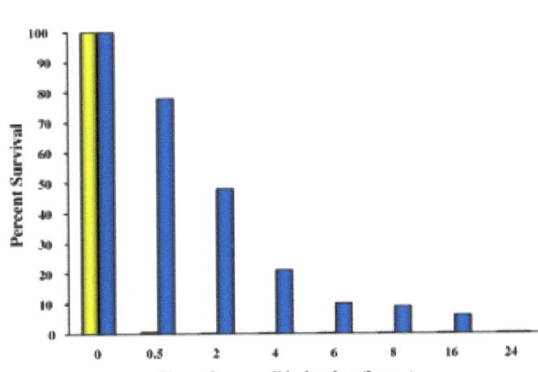

B.

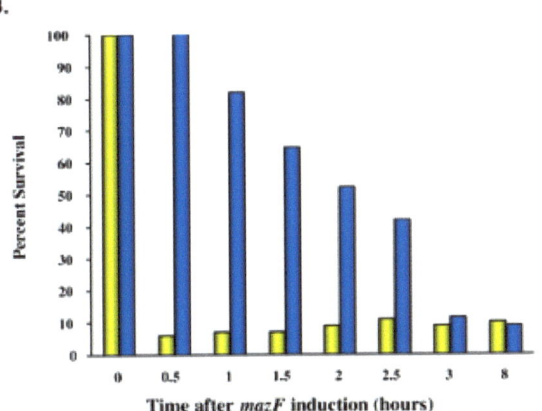

ABSTRACT

Tracheary elements (TEs) have a unique cell death program in which the rapid collapse of the vacuole triggers the beginning of nuclear degradation. Although various nucleases are known to function in nuclear DNA degradation in animal apoptosis, it is unclear what hydrolase is involved in nuclear degradation in plants. In this study, we demonstrated that an S1-type nuclease, Zinnia endonuclease 1 (ZEN1), functions directly in nuclear DNA degradation during programmed cell death (PCD) of TEs. In-gel DNase assay demonstrated the presence of a 24-kD Ca^{2+}/Mg^{2+}-dependent nuclease and a 40-kD Zn^{2+}-dependent nuclease as well as ZEN1 in 60-h-cultured cells that included differentiating TEs. Such cell extracts possessed the ability to degrade the nuclear DNA isolated from *Zinnia elegans* cells in the presence of Zn^{2+}, and its activity was suppressed by an anti-ZEN1 antibody, indicating that ZEN1 is a central DNase responsible for nuclear DNA degradation. The introduction of the antisense *ZEN1* gene into Zinnia cells cultured for 40 h specifically suppressed the degradation of nuclear DNA in TEs undergoing PCD but did not affect vacuole collapse. Based on these results, a common mechanism between animal and plant PCD is discussed.

INTRODUCTION

In most multicellular organisms, programmed cell death (PCD) is built into the processes of normal development and growth. One key event in PCD is DNA degradation, because the degradation of the genome is considered to be a means by which the cell death program is made irreversible and facilitates the disassembly of the nucleus. Indeed, DNA degradation is a hallmark of apoptosis during PCD in animal cells (Wyllie, 1980; Jacobson et al., 1997). Apoptotic DNA degradation occurs in at least three stages (Wyllie, 1980; Oberhammer et al., 1993). Early in the process, DNA is cleaved to high molecular mass fragments (50 to 200 kb) consistent with the size of chromatin loop domains. The subsequent cleavage of DNA occurs at the internucleosomal linker region, and its products produce a 180-bp DNA ladder. Importantly, some cell lines exhibit only high molecular mass DNA cleavage (Oberhammer et al., 1993). Finally, the fragmented DNA in apoptotic cells is digested completely by an enzyme(s) such as DNase II produced by engulfing cells (McIlroy et al., 2000). To date, apoptosis-inducing factor (Susin et al., 1999), topoisomerase II (Li et al., 1999), and caspase-activated DFF/CAD-ICAD (Sakahira et al., 1999) have been implicated in the early process of DNA cleavage. On the other hand, internucleosomal cleavage is known to be associated with several endonucleases, including caspase-activated

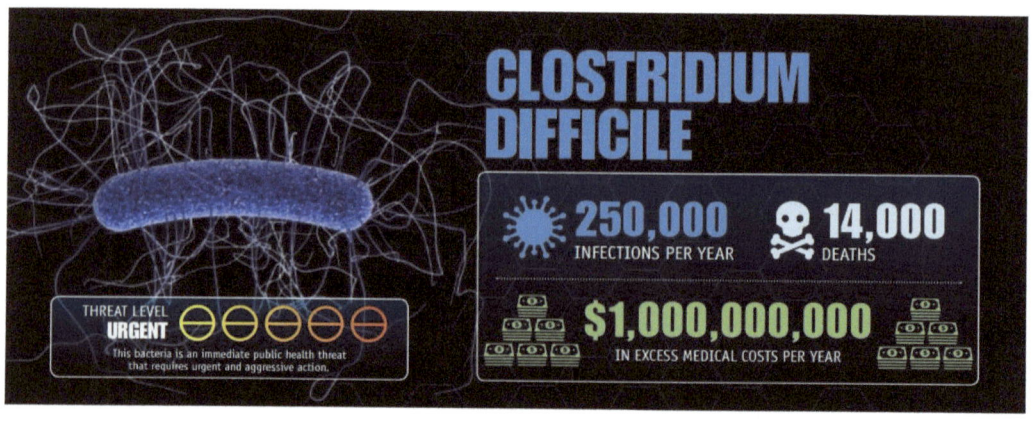

Gene mutations that can lead to cancer

The 2 main types of genes that play a role in cancer are *oncogenes* and *tumor suppressor genes*.

Oncogenes

Most oncogenes are mutations of certain normal genes called *proto-oncogenes*. Proto-oncogenes are the "good" genes that normally control what kind of cell it is and how often it divides. When a proto-oncogene mutates (changes) into an oncogene, it becomes a "bad" gene that can become permanently turned on or activated when it is not supposed to be. When this happens, the cell grows out of control, which can lead to cancer.

It may be helpful to think of a cell as a car. For it to work properly, there need to be ways to control how fast it goes. A proto-oncogene normally functions in a way that is much like a gas pedal. It helps the cell grow and divide. An oncogene could be compared with a gas pedal that is stuck down, which causes the cell to divide out of control.

As scientists learn more about oncogenes, they may be able to develop drugs that inhibit or stop them. Some drugs that target oncogenes are already being used, and more are on the way. This is discussed in more detail later on in this document.

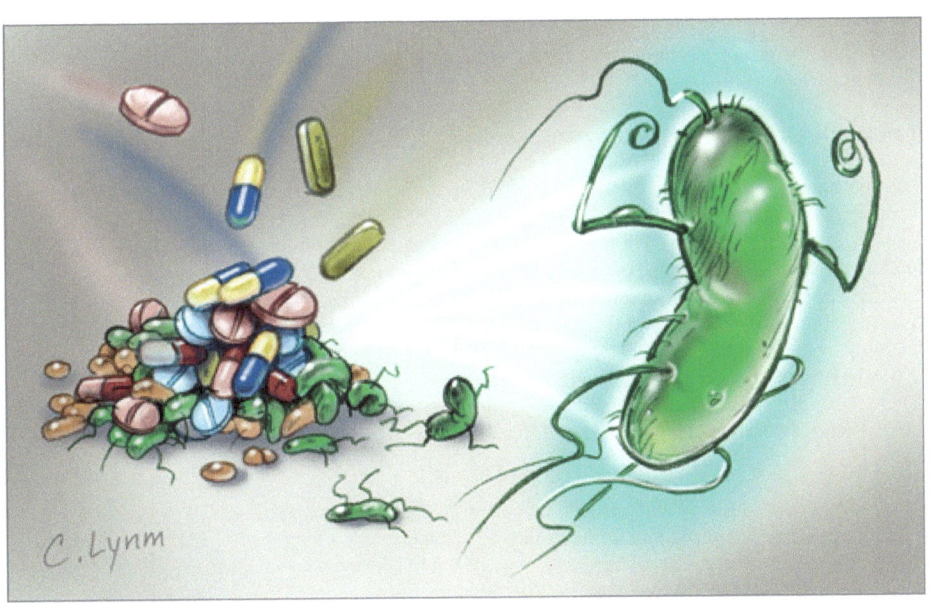

C. Lynm

Inherited mutations of oncogenes

A few cancer syndromes are caused by inherited mutations of proto-oncogenes that cause the oncogene to be turned on (activated). For example, multiple endocrine neoplasia type 2 (MEN2) is caused by an inherited mutation in the gene called *RET*. People affected by this syndrome often develop an uncommon thyroid cancer called medullary cancer of the thyroid. They also develop other tumors, including pheochromocytoma and nerve tumors. Inherited mutations in the gene called *KIT* can cause hereditary gastrointestinal stromal tumors (GISTs). And inherited mutations in the gene called *MET* can cause hereditary papillary renal cancer.

Acquired mutations of oncogenes

Most cancer-causing mutations involving oncogenes are acquired, not inherited. They generally activate oncogenes by chromosome rearrangements, gene duplication, or mutation. For example, a chromosome rearrangement can lead to formation of the gene called *BCR-ABL*, which leads to chronic myeloid leukemia (CML). Acquired mutations that activate the *KIT* gene cause most cases of gastrointestinal stromal tumor (GIST).

Tumor suppressor genes

Tumor suppressor genes are normal genes that slow down cell division, repair DNA mistakes, or tell cells when to die (a process known as *apoptosis* or *programmed cell death*). When tumor suppressor genes don't work properly, cells can grow out of control, which can lead to cancer. Many different tumor suppressor genes have been found, including *TP53 (p53)*, *BRCA1*, *BRCA2*, *APC*, and *RB1*.

A tumor suppressor gene is like the brake pedal on a car. It normally keeps the cell from dividing too quickly, just as a brake keeps a car from going too fast. When something goes wrong with the gene, such as a mutation, cell division can get out of control.

An important difference between oncogenes and tumor suppressor genes is that oncogenes result from the *activation* (turning on) of proto-oncogenes, but tumor suppressor genes cause cancer when they are *inactivated* (turned off).

Inherited mutations of tumor suppressor genes

Inherited abnormalities of tumor suppressor genes have been found in some family cancer syndromes. They cause certain types of cancer to run in families. For example, a defective *APC* gene causes *familial adenomatous polyposis (FAP)*, a condition in which people develop hundreds or even thousands of colon polyps. Often, at least one of the polyps becomes cancer, leading to colon cancer. There are many examples of inherited tumor suppressor gene mutations, and more are being discovered each year. For more information about inherited mutations and cancer, see our document *Heredity and Cancer*.

Acquired mutations of tumor suppressor genes

Tumor suppressor gene mutations have been found in many cancers. Most of these mutations are acquired, not inherited.

For example, abnormalities of the *TP53* gene (which codes for the p53 protein) have been found in more than half of human cancers. Acquired mutations of this gene appear in a wide range of cancers, including lung, colorectal, and breast cancer. The p53 protein is involved in the pathway to apoptosis. This pathway is turned on when a cell has DNA damage that can't be repaired. If the gene for p53 is not working properly, cells with damaged DNA continue to grow and divide. Over time this can lead to cancer.

Acquired changes in many other tumor suppressor genes also contribute to the development of sporadic (not inherited) cancers.

A little Anthropology

Sex with Neanderthals had its ups and its downs. Cross-breeding may have given modern humans genes useful for coping with climates colder than Africa's, but the hybrid offspring probably suffered from significant fertility problems.

Those conclusions come from two papers published today in *Science*[1] and *Nature*[2], which identify the slices of the genome that contemporary humans inherited from Neanderthals, the stocky hunter-gatherers that went extinct around 30,000 years ago.

Homo sapiens and Neanderthals share a common ancestor that probably lived in Africa more than half a million years ago. The ancestors of Neanderthals were the first to move to Europe and Asia while the modern-human lineage stayed in Africa. But after modern humans began to leave Africa less than 100,000 years ago, they interbred with the Neanderthals who had settled on a range stretching from Western Europe to Siberia.

"These were bits of the genomes that had not seen each other for half a million years," says David Reich, a population geneticist at Harvard Medical School in Boston, Massachusetts, who led the *Nature* study along with colleague Sriram Sankararaman. "That's something that doesn't happen in human populations today."

The magic number

Genome sequences harvested from Neanderthal bones have previously confirmed that the two groups mated, and that about 2% of the genomes of people who descend from Europeans, Asians and other non-Africans is Neanderthal[3,4]. The Neanderthal contributions are peppered across the genome, and different people have different Neanderthal genes.

BMC
Musculoskeletal Disorders

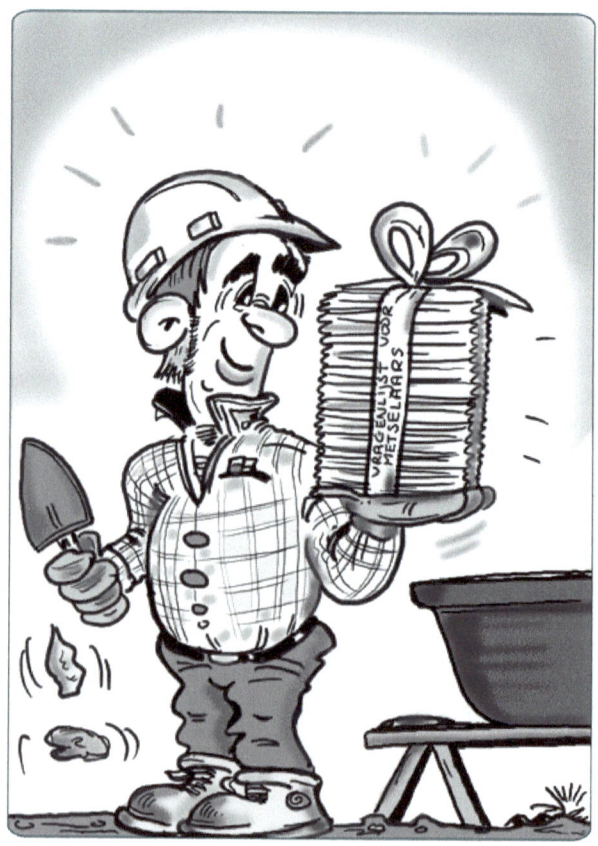

Musculoskeletal disorders among construction workers: a one-year follow-up study

Boschman *et al.*

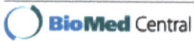

Boschman *et al. BMC Musculoskeletal Disorders* 2012, **13**:196
http://www.biomedcentral.com/1471-2474/13/196

Related stories

Research has indicated that some of these genes are involved in functions such as battling infections[5, 6] and coping with ultraviolet radiation[7]. But the latest studies are the first to identify a large proportion of the genome segments that humans inherited from Neanderthals.

Both teams developed computational methods to identify segments of the human genome that were likely to have originated hundreds of thousands of years in the past, yet entered the human gene pool far more recently. The teams then checked whether or not these segments were present in the actual Neanderthal genome sequence to come up with a catalog of Neanderthal genes in humans.

Joshua Akey, a population geneticist at the University of Washington in Seattle who wrote the *Science* paper with colleague Benjamin Vernot, says that his team found about one-fifth of a Neanderthal genome spread across the publicly available genomes of 665 living Europeans and East Asians. Reich and his team estimate that they could put together about 40% of the Neanderthal genome from the sequences of 1,004 living people that they studied.

The teams looked for Neanderthal genes that were especially common in contemporary humans, a sign that the genes were useful to their new owners. Both groups identified a series of genes involved in the inner workings of cells called keratinocytes, which make up most of the outer layer of human skin and produce hair.

"It's tempting to speculate that Neanderthals were already adapted to colder environments in Eurasia" and that these genes helped modern humans to cope after they arrived from Africa, says Reich. Akey points out that the skin helps to mediate moisture loss and protect against pathogens, and Neanderthal genes that were already adapted to life in Europe and Asia would be helpful to *H. sapiens* in its new environment. These hypotheses are speculative, the researchers say, and they agree that follow-up studies will be needed to determine how Neanderthal keratinocyte genes benefited modern humans.

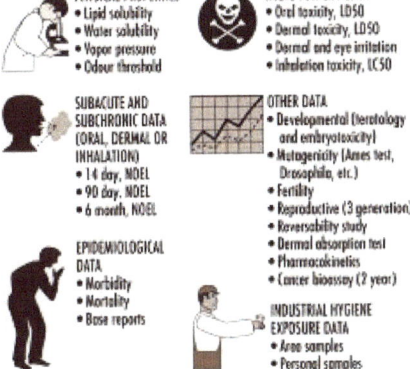

Both studies also discovered vast numbers of Neanderthal genes that none of the contemporary humans carried. "We find these gigantic holes in the human genomes where there are no surviving Neanderthal lineages," says Akey. This is a strong indication that the genes were harmful to human–Neanderthal hybrids and their descendants, and were purged as the descendants continued to mate. "Most of these variations were removed in a couple of dozen generations," Reich says.

Akey's team found that one large chunk of modern-human genome that bears no Neanderthal contributions is the one that encompasses the gene *FOXP2*, which is involved in speech in humans.

Mixed messages

Reich's team, meanwhile, discovered that today's humans tend to have few of the Neanderthal genes that are activated in the testes or located on the X chromosome. In organisms such as fruitflies, such patterns are hallmarks of hybrid sterility, indicating that two populations are too distantly related to breed successfully. Modern humans and Neanderthals "were at the edge of biological compatibility", Reich concludes, and their hybrids probably suffered high rates of infertility.

"Neanderthals aren't around, so you can't do a mating experiment," says Daven Presgraves, an evolutionary biologist at the University of Rochester in New York. But the patterns that Reich's team noticed are exactly what you would expect if their hybrids suffered from reduced fertility, he adds.

However, Presgraves was surprised that modern humans and Neanderthals, separated by only tens of thousands of generations, would already show signs biological incompatibility. Animals such as fruitflies typically need to be separated for much longer to evolve naturally into distinct species, he says.

Sarah Tishkoff, a population geneticist at the University of Pennsylvania in Philadelphia, says that the studies rank as "some of the most exciting papers I've seen". She adds that the work hints at the possibility of studying ancient-human genomes gleaned not from bones but from the DNA of contemporary populations.

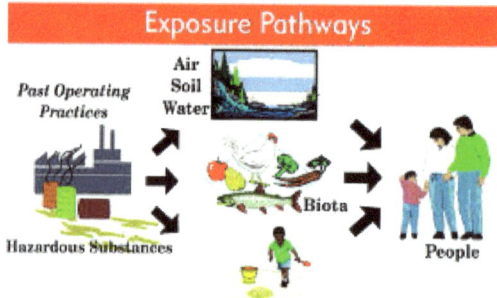

Such studies could be especially revealing in Africa (see 'African genes tracked back'). There, well-preserved samples of ancient DNA are scarce, and yet genome studies of today's inhabitants of the continent[8] hints that although ancient Africans did not mingle with Neanderthals they may have interbred with other now-extinct groups. "We really need to be able to apply these methods to African populations," says Tishkoff. "Just imagine what we're going to find there."

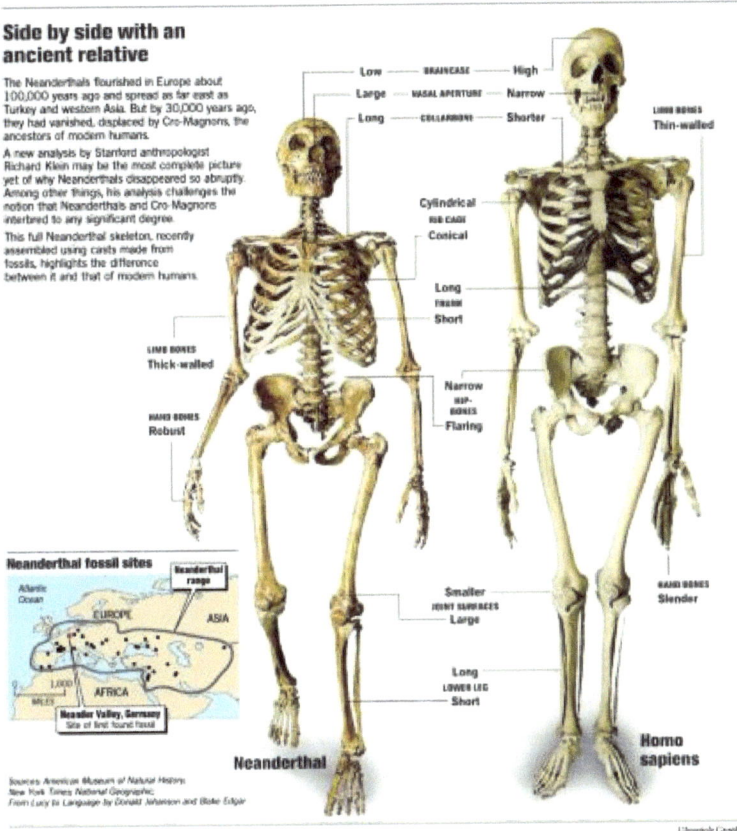

Side by side with an ancient relative

The Neanderthals flourished in Europe about 100,000 years ago and spread as far east as Turkey and western Asia. But by 30,000 years ago, they had vanished, displaced by Cro-Magnons, the ancestors of modern humans.

A new analysis by Stanford anthropologist Richard Klein may be the most complete picture yet of why Neanderthals disappeared so abruptly. Among other things, his analysis challenges the notion that Neanderthals and Cro-Magnons interbred to any significant degree.

This full Neanderthal skeleton, recently assembled using casts made from fossils, highlights the difference between it and that of modern humans.

BRAINCASE — Low ... High
NASAL APERTURE — Large ... Narrow
COLLARBONE — Long ... Shorter
LIMB BONES Thin-walled

RIB CAGE — Cylindrical ... Conical

FEMUR — Long ... Short

LIMB BONES Thick-walled

HIP BONES — Narrow ... Flaring

HAND BONES Robust

HAND BONES Slender

JOINT SURFACES — Smaller ... Large

LOWER LEG — Long ... Short

Neanderthal fossil sites

Neanderthal range

Atlantic Ocean
EUROPE
ASIA
AFRICA
1,000 MILES

Neander Valley, Germany
Site of first found fossil

Sources: American Museum of Natural History; New York Times; National Geographic; From Lucy to Language by Donald Johanson and Blake Edgar

Neanderthal

Homo sapiens

Another ancient genome, another mystery. DNA gleaned from a 400,000-year-old femur from Spain has revealed an unexpected link between Europe's hominin inhabitants of the time and a cryptic population, the Denisovans, who are known to have lived much more recently in southwestern Siberia.

- 'Atomtronic' superfluid remembers how it has been stirred
- Genome of 'Clovis boy' raises questions on handling of Native American remains
- UK reveals decontamination procedures for terror attacks

The DNA, which represents the oldest hominin sequence yet published, has left researchers baffled because most of them believed that the bones would be more closely linked to Neanderthals than to Denisovans. "That's not what I would have expected;

that's not what anyone would have expected," says Chris Stringer, a palaeoanthropologist at London's Natural History Museum who was not involved in sequencing the femur DNA.

The fossil was excavated in the 1990s from a deep cave in a well-studied site in northern Spain called Sima de los Huesos ('pit of bones'). This femur and the remains of more than two dozen other hominins found at the site have previously been attributed either to early forms of Neanderthals, who lived in Europe until about 30,000 years ago, or to *Homo heidelbergensis*, a loosely defined hominin population that gave rise to Neanderthals in Europe and possibly humans in Africa.

But a closer link to Neanderthals than to Denisovans was not what was discovered by the team led by Svante Pääbo, a molecular geneticist at the Max Planck Institute for Evolutionary Anthropology in Leipzig, Germany.

Listen

Svante Pääbo talks to Ewen Callaway about the hominin DNA

`00:00`

The team sequenced most of the femur's mitochondrial genome, which is made up of DNA from the cell's energy-producing structures and passed down the maternal line. The resulting phylogenetic analysis — which shows branches in evolutionary history — placed the DNA closer to that of Denisovans than to Neanderthals or modern humans. "This really raises more questions than it answers," Pääbo says.

The team's finding, published online in *Nature* this week, does not necessarily mean that the Sima de los Huesos hominins are more closely related to the Denisovans, a population that lived thousands of kilometres away and hundreds of thousands of years later, than to nearby Neanderthals. This is because the mitochondrial genome tells the history of just an individual's mother, and her mother, and so on.

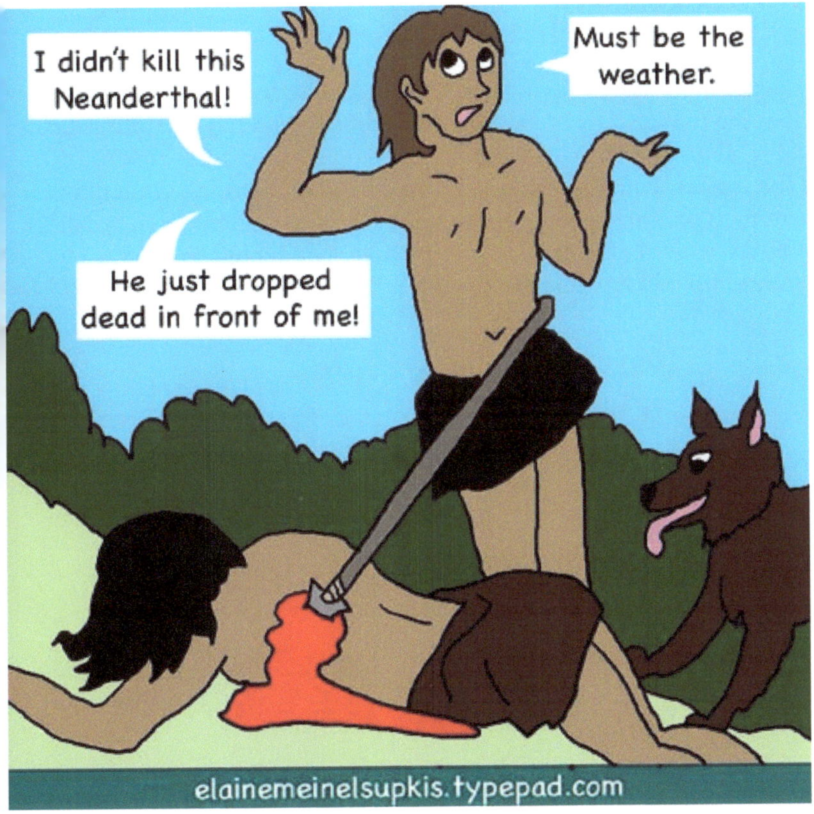

FAMILY MYSTERY

The mitochondrial genome of a 400,000-year-old femur has an unexpected link with a group of hominins called Denisovans. One interpretation is that this could be the result of interbreeding between more ancient populations, such as *Homo antecessor* and *Homo heidelbergensis*.

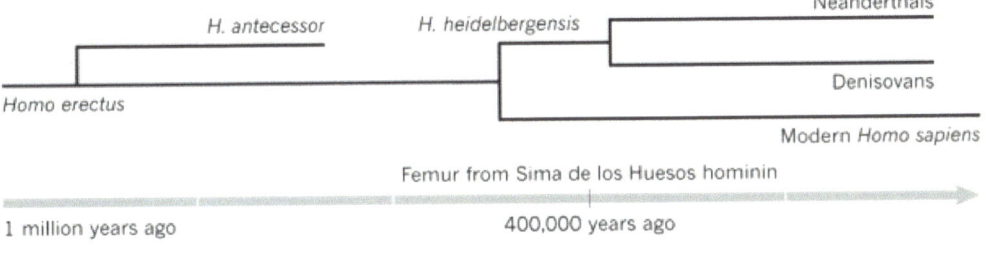

Expand

Nuclear DNA, by contrast, contains material from both parents (and all of their ancestors) and typically provides a more accurate overview of a population's history. But this was not available from the femur.

With that caveat in mind, researchers interested in human evolution are scrambling to explain the surprising link, and everyone seems to have their own ideas.

Pääbo notes that previously published full nuclear genomes of Neanderthals and Denisovans suggest that the two had a common ancestor that lived up to 700,000 years ago. He suggests that the Sima de los Huesos hominins could represent a founder population that once lived all over Eurasia and gave rise to the two groups. Both may have then carried the mitochondrial sequence seen in the caves. But these mitochondrial lineages go extinct whenever a female does not give birth to a daughter, so the Neanderthals could have simply lost that sequence while it lived on in Denisovan women.

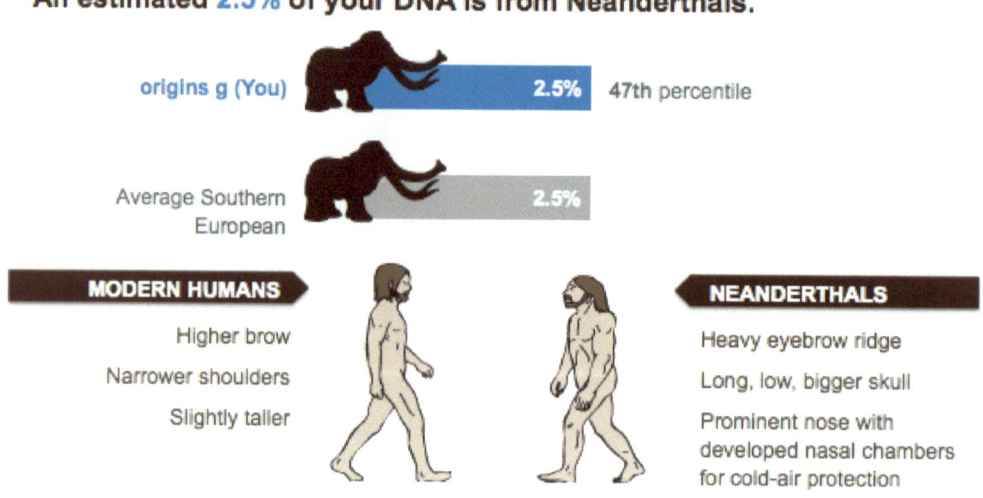

An estimated 2.5% of your DNA is from Neanderthals.

origins g (You) — 2.5% — 47th percentile

Average Southern European — 2.5%

MODERN HUMANS
Higher brow
Narrower shoulders
Slightly taller

NEANDERTHALS
Heavy eyebrow ridge
Long, low, bigger skull
Prominent nose with developed nasal chambers for cold-air protection

"I've got my own twist on it," says Stringer, who has previously argued that the Sima de los Huesos hominins are indeed early Neanderthals (C. Stringer *Evol. Anthropol.* **21,** 101–107; 2012). He thinks that the newly decoded mitochondrial genome may have come from another distinct group of hominins. Not far from the caves, researchers have discovered hominin bones from about 800,000 years ago that have been attributed to an archaic hominin called *Homo antecessor*, thought to be a European descendant of *Homo erectus*. Stringer proposes that this species interbred with a population that was ancestral to both Denisovans and Sima de los Huesos hominins, introducing the newly decoded mitochondrial lineage to both populations (see 'Family mystery').

This scenario, Stringer says, explains another oddity thrown up by the sequencing of ancient hominin DNA. As part of a widely discussed and soon-to-be-released analysis of high-quality Denisovan and Neanderthal nuclear genomes, Pääbo's team suggests that Denisovans seem to have interbred with a mysterious hominin group.

The situation will become clearer if Pääbo's team can eke nuclear DNA out of the bones from the Sima de los Huesos hominins, which his team hopes to achieve within a year or so.

Obtaining such sequences will not be simple, because nuclear DNA is present in bone at much lower levels than mitochondrial DNA. And even obtaining the partial mitochondrial genome was not easy: the team had to grind up almost two grams of bone and relied on various technical and computational methods to sequence the contaminated and damaged DNA and to arrange it into a genome. To make sure that they had identified genuine ancient sequences, they analysed only very short DNA strands that contained chemical modifications characteristic of ancient DNA.

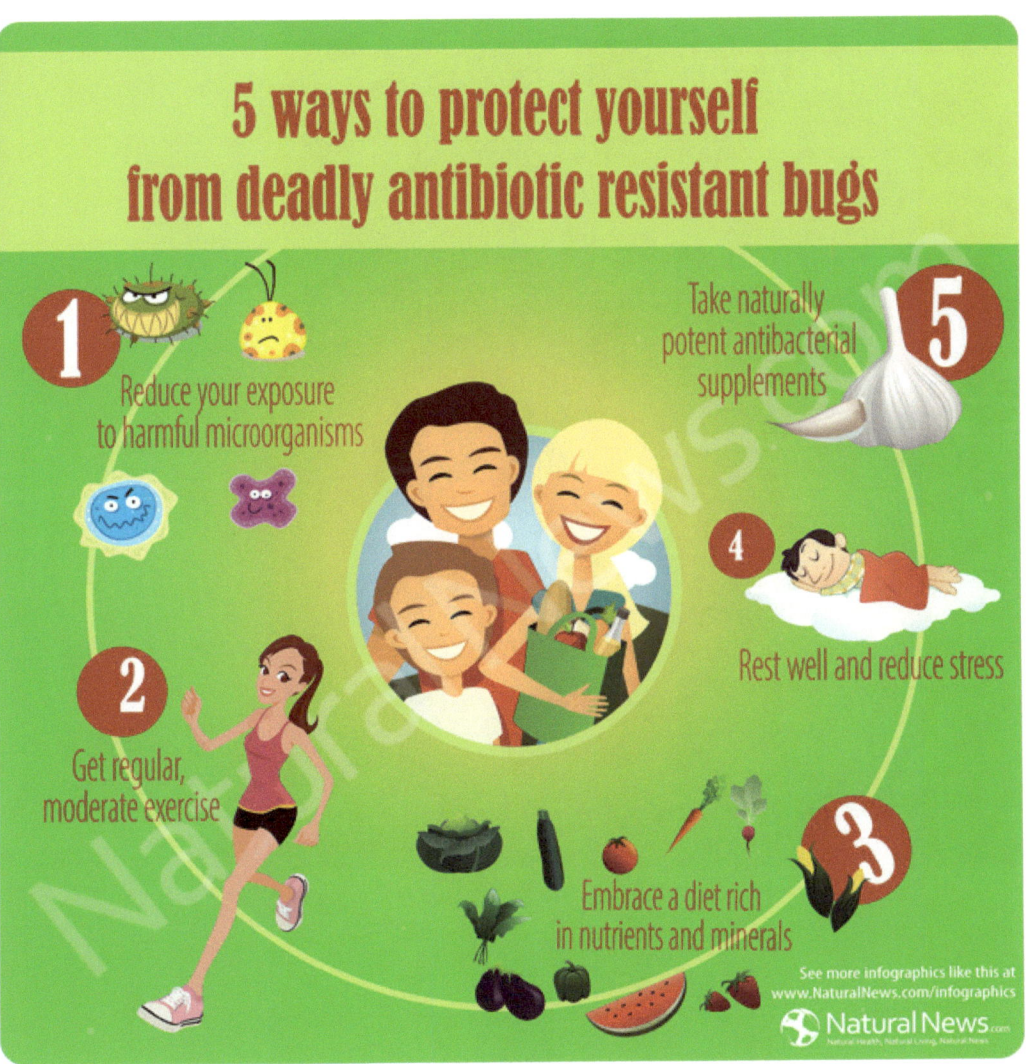

A Healthy Lifestyle with lots of fresh air, healthy food cooked in a clean environment, little exposure and routine practices can prevent further proliferations of germs in the environment, hospitals and in public areas.

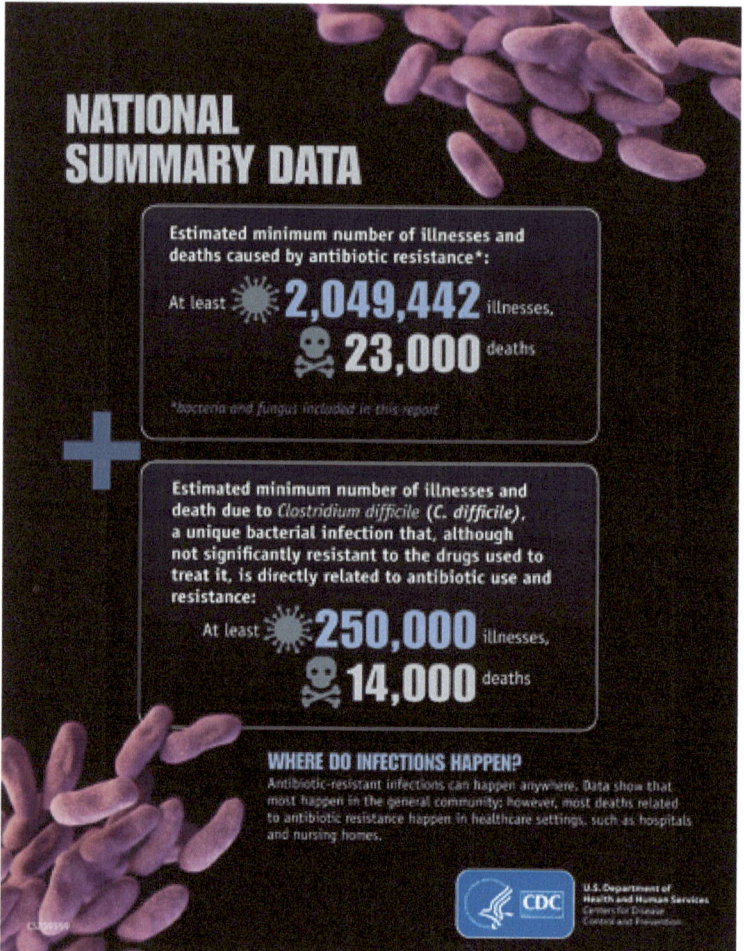

NATIONAL SUMMARY DATA

Estimated minimum number of illnesses and deaths caused by antibiotic resistance*:

At least **2,049,442** illnesses,
23,000 deaths

*bacteria and fungus included in this report

Estimated minimum number of illnesses and death due to *Clostridium difficile* (*C. difficile*), a unique bacterial infection that, although not significantly resistant to the drugs used to treat it, is directly related to antibiotic use and resistance:

At least **250,000** illnesses,
14,000 deaths

WHERE DO INFECTIONS HAPPEN?

Antibiotic-resistant infections can happen anywhere. Data show that most happen in the general community; however, most deaths related to antibiotic resistance happen in healthcare settings, such as hospitals and nursing homes.

CDC — U.S. Department of Health and Human Services, Centers for Disease Control and Prevention

www.ingramcontent.com/pod-product-compliance
Lightning Source LLC
Chambersburg PA
CBHW042240290526
45792CB00021B/935